ASPERGERS
SYNDROME

The Easy-to-understand and Practical Guide for
Parents

(Making Way for Asperger's Syndrome)

Debbra Prince

Published by Tomas Edwards

© **Debbra Prince**

All Rights Reserved

Aspergers Syndrome: The Easy-to-understand and Practical Guide for Parents (Making Way for Asperger's Syndrome)

ISBN 978-1-990268-72-4

Legal & Disclaimer

The information contained in this book is not designed to replace or take the place of any form of medicine or professional medical advice. The information in this book has been provided for educational and entertainment purposes only.

The information contained in this book has been compiled from sources deemed reliable, and it is accurate to the best of the Author's knowledge; however, the Author cannot guarantee its accuracy and validity and cannot be held liable for any errors or omissions. Changes are periodically made to this book. You must consult your doctor or get professional medical advice before using any of the suggested remedies, techniques, or information in this book.

Table of Contents

INTRODUCTION...1

CHAPTER 1: ASPERGER'S SYNDROME EXPLAINED 2

CHAPTER 2: THERAPIES 28

CHAPTER 3: COMPASSIONATE UNDERSTANDING OF THE ASPERGER ADULT..34

CHAPTER 4: IT A-S HOW YOU SEE IT 39

CHAPTER 5: EFFECTS OF THE SYNDROME ON SOCIAL INTERACTION 47

CHAPTER 6: ASPERGER'S SYNDROME AND SOCIAL INTERACTION 66

CONCLUSION..89

Introduction

Asperger's Syndrome is also called PDD, a group of conditions in which many basic skills are delayed, most commonly the ability to socialize with others, communication skills, and imaginative ability.

Although Asperger's Syndrome resembles Autism (one of the most severe types of PDD) in a number of ways, there are major differences that distinguish the two. Asperger's children commonly function at a higher level than autistic children. In addition, Asperger's Syndrome children have near-average intelligence, and development of language that is near to normal, which may be increased with the passage of time.

The disorder was named after an Austrian doctor named Hans Asperger, who described this disorder for the first time in 1944. Though until much later Asperger's Syndrome was not known as distinctive disorder.

1

Chapter 1: Asperger's Syndrome Explained

It was a typical Saturday morning when 6-year old Simon and his parents sat down at the waiting room of Dr. Lassen's clinic. Simon's parents finally decided to take him to a specialist after considering the concerns that were brought up by Simon's teachers. His teachers have observed that Simon's behavior at school was very unpredictable and inconsistent. They have also noticed that there would be times when he would suddenly show an intense stream of emotion. They observed him closely after a few outbursts thinking that the child is just showing tantrums. He also showed difficulties with maintaining eye contact. However, the thing that convinced them that there was indeed something strange with Simon's behavior when he started inflicting harm to himself. He would often pinch himself or bang his head on the wall. Both his parents and teachers thought that Simon was just a hyperactive kid that preferred playing alone which is why they were astonished when the psychologist diagnosed him with Asperger's Syndrome.

During the initial observation and assessment of Simon, it was found that he had attention disorder, general learning disabilities, as well as impairments with his perception and processing of information. His mother reported that she became ill during the first trimester of her pregnancy with him. The doctors found no problems or complications with Simon during his first few weeks as an infant. However, when he was about 11 months old, his parents noticed that although he was already walking and running, he had difficulties with his speech. They assumed that Simon was speech delayed. They also observed that his fine motor skills were underdeveloped. He had difficulties with accomplishing simple tasks such as properly holding utensils, brushing his hair, dressing up as well as climbing up and down the stairs.

After an in depth evaluation and assessment of Simon, the doctor recommended a treatment program that targeted the specific difficulties that Simon was experiencing. Through the series of tests given to him, they were able to pin point the factors that were contributing to his behavior. For instance, they detected that Simon had a weak connection between the hemispheres of his brain. They also found disturbances and deficiencies with his vestibular, auditory, visual, and tactile sensitivities. When these problems were addressed, they were able to design a comprehensive intervention program for him. Through treatment and therapy, Simon was given more opportunities to learn, grow and live life to fullest. His teachers also noticed that he had improvements with his behavior in the classroom. He was starting to relate with his classmates better. His mood became more positive and the occurrence of his tantrums greatly decreased. As you can see, the proper diagnosis, treatment and intervention significantly improved the behavior of Simon both at home and at school.

Overview

In 2014, the Centers for Disease Control and Prevention (CDC) reported that the estimated prevalence of Autism Spectrum Disorder in the United States alone occur in about 1 in 68 births; which means that approximately 3.5 million Americans are diagnosed with autism. Autism Spectrum Disorder or ASD is characterized by a wide range of symptoms that differ in degree or severity. People with ASD that fall under the lower end of the spectrum (lower functioning) are usually diagnosed with autistic disorder. However, people belonging to the higher side of the spectrum are identified with having Asperger's Syndrome and are considered to be high functioning individuals that only require substantial support. This book is focused primarily on raising the awareness of its readers about the less severe form of autism or more commonly known as Asperger's Syndrome.

Since ASD is one of the most unpredictable and wide ranged developmental disorders, it is also one of the most frequently misunderstood conditions that have a direct impact on the life of an individual. In fact, a lot of people enter adulthood and live their lives without even getting a formal diagnosis of their condition. These individuals are almost always "assumed" to just be socially awkward with poor social and communication skills as well as having their "own" unique way of thinking and behaving. A lot of them are labeled as "eccentric", "strange", and even naughty.

Autism vs. Asperger's Syndrome

The primary difference between Autism and Asperger's Syndrome is the severity of the symptoms. Children with Asperger's usually have average communication and cognitive skills. From a typical person's perspective, they may seem like a normal child, but with strange or odd behavior.

Also, children with lower functioning Autism usually act awkwardly in social situations. Children with Asperger's on the other hand, want to interact with others, but do not know how to do it.

Another significant difference between the two is that people with Asperger's usually don't have speech delays. But, they may still express unusual speech patterns and have difficulties with understanding the subtleties of language. Their motor skills are not as severe as those with lower functioning autism, but they may still seem awkward or clumsy.

"Dash of Autism"

In 1940, a Pediatrician named Hans Asperger discovered distinct behaviors from certain males and females and compared them with the communication and social skills of people of normal intelligence. Some professionals described this condition as a milder form of Autism. They used the term "high-functioning Autism". On the other hand, a professor from the Institute of Cognitive Neuroscience at the University College London named Uta Frith also described this disorder as "having a dash of autism".

The condition is more common in males than in females. Not unless a child shows some serious difficulties in their personal lives, school or workplace, Asperger's Syndrome will generally remain undiagnosed. Asperger's Syndrome is probably underdiagnosed, but at least 2-3 persons of every 1000 people in the United States have this condition. Families may often think that the symptoms shown by their child are related to depression or anxiety.

For a normal person, when you meet someone, you have to use a proper tone of voice and gestures in communicating, which are observed and learned over time. However, for a person diagnosed with Asperger's Syndrome, these skills are very difficult to do. They can communicate, but most of the topics will focus on only one topic and they often lack social interaction.

Considering all these, Asperger's Syndrome was included in the American Psychiatric Association's Diagnostic and Statistical Manual of Mental Disorders in

1994. Asperger's Syndrome is considered a disorder under Autism Spectrum Disorder.

For some reason, others may think that a person with Asperger's Syndrome is just afraid to mix with other people or is just not interested in sharing ideas with others. Asperger's Disorder is usually diagnosed when the child levels up in secondary school or when there are certain changes in the environment that requires them to adjust.

Causes

Until today, experts cannot pin point the exact factors that cause Asperger's syndrome. Since Asperger's is considered to be a milder form of Autism, its causes are quite similar with that of Autism. Experts believe that both environmental and biological factors increase the likelihood of the development of the condition.

Additionally, other factors that may affect the development of this syndrome are environmental toxins such as viruses or chemicals, and genetic factors. However, physicians are still looking for the exact cause of this disorder.

Environmental Factors

Researchers believe that there are a lot of possible causes for a person to have Asperger's Syndrome. The consensus among researchers states that environmental factors play a vital role with exacerbation of Autism symptoms.

a. Vaccines

Some parents even say that they just become aware of Autism after the routine vaccination of the child. However, there is no scientific evidence that would prove it. It may also be due to genetic factors, but the studies are incomplete to prove this possible cause.

b. Prenatal Development

Some people also say that Autism is somewhat associated with the prenatal environment and development. The prenatal factors include diabetes, bleeding, advanced aged parents, and psychiatric medications during the first 8 weeks of pregnancy. However, these cases are rare and there is no evidence that would prove if these factors are true.

Additionally, it has been hypothesized that folic acid and prenatal stress may also cause Autism. But the research is incomplete. Further, as per fetal testosterone theory, there is a belief that the high level of testosterone pushes the brain development leading to broad and complex cognitive skills while diminishing empathy and communication skills. However, these studies are not supported by scientific evidences.

c. Exposure to Toxins

There are postnatal environmental factors affecting formation of Autism as well, although these factors are not yet confirmed. Some of these factors include gastrointestinal or immune system abnormalities, allergies, and exposure to drugs such as opioids, vaccines, infection, certain foods, or heavy metals. These evidences were not yet confirmed by research.

Moreover, when it comes to foods, researchers indicate that Vitamin D deficiency may also cause Autism. However, this was not yet proven. Lead blood levels of children with Autism are high. Therefore, researchers believe that this has something to do with lead poisoning. Mercury poisoning is also believed to be one of the factors that may cause Autism, as the symptoms of a child experiencing Mercury poisoning is the same with a child that has Autism. Still, the evidence was not enough to prove this study.

Biological Factors

It is also believed that genetic factors play a significant role in the development of Asperger's syndrome. Multiple genes were found to have contributed to causing this condition which is why some experts consider that genetics is a principal cause of Asperger's syndrome

Identical twin studies increase the possibility that there are certain genes responsible for the development of this condition. Although no particular gene has been identified to cause Autism, research suggests that genes still play an important role in its development. It is supposed that patients with no family history of Autism may have developed the condition because of certain gene mutations.

The studies, researches, surveys and myths presented still lack enough scientific evidence that would show accuracy. Asperger's Syndrome is a developmental disorder considered to be an Autism Spectrum Disorder. There may be a lot of factors that may possibly contribute to its development, but the direct and main causes of this condition remain unknown.

Definition and General Information about Asperger's Syndrome

☐ Asperger's Syndrome was discovered by a Pediatrician named Hans Asperger in 1940.

☐ Asperger's Syndrome is a developmental disorder, not an illness or a disease.

☐ Asperger's Syndrome is known as "having a dash of Autism," or a milder form of Autism.

☐ The main cause is unclear. Researchers show that this condition may be due to genetic and neurological factors, autoimmune diseases, prenatal and postnatal environmental factors, vaccines, toxins, and lack of parental affection. These factors still lack enough scientific evidence.

□ According to The World Health Organization, there are more males being diagnosed with this disorder than females.

□ Asperger's Syndrome is usually diagnosed late due to similar symptoms with other disorders, including Attention Deficit Hyperactivity Disorder, Schizophrenia, and Obsessive-Compulsive Disorder.

Symptoms and Diagnosis

A person with Asperger's Syndrome may be diagnosed with a wrong condition such as Schizophrenia, Attention Deficit Hyperactivity Disorder, Anxiety or Depression due to the similarity of the symptoms. Some people with Asperger's Syndrome are good at hiding their difficulties or weaknesses, which include the inability to interact well with other people, inability to understand body language, inability to imagine things and possible solutions, inability to give up repetitive behaviors or routines, and the inability to do motor skills properly.

Hiding all these difficulties are not easy. The affected person might feel rejected, exhausted, uncomfortable, uneasy, confused, sad and weak due to the pressure of having Asperger's Syndrome. These weaknesses may even lead to a more serious type of depression. This is one of the reasons why they always choose to be alone: to get away from possible discrimination and possible insults. They are intelligent and some of them even attain an above-average intelligence. They have great thinking abilities.

The best way to manage Asperger's syndrome is early diagnosis and treatment. If you are noticing that your child or someone you know is displaying peculiar behaviors, do not hesitate to consult with a professional. Familiarizing yourself with the symptoms of Asperger's syndrome will allow you to anticipate the unpredictable behavior and not confuse Asperger's Syndrome with other disorders.

Symptoms

As I have mentioned in this book earlier, Asperger's syndrome is considered to be a "dash of Autism" because of the fact that people with this condition have average to above average intelligence, language, and cognitive skills. This is why some people with this condition can grow old without even getting a formal diagnosis. To prevent this from happening, here are the common symptoms of Asperger's Syndrome:

a. Difficulties with Social Interactions

People who are diagnosed with Asperger's Syndrome may exhibit limited social interactions. Some common traits include minimal eye contact, robotic or repetitive speech, and difficulty interpreting non-verbal communication such as gestures and facial expressions. There is a tendency to lack an understanding for emotional issues, but then again, this can be gradually improved with social programs and treatments, which will be discussed later. For some time, a person with this condition may try to have some friends, but may lose connection due to their poor social skills. As a result, they may just choose to stay alone.

b. They may lack Empathy

A person with Asperger's Syndrome may not respond with a smile or a nod, or may not make eye contact when talking to someone. Additionally, they may not understand the usual flow of a conversation. They may also be unaware of the appropriate action at a certain place. For example, when you enter a private room in a hospital to visit a sick friend or when inside the church, the affected person may speak too loudly without even observing silence as a sign of respect whenever inside these places. They may also lack emotional instinct. For example, a friend is sharing a sad story and suddenly cries. The person with Asperger's Syndrome may not understand why they are crying, so they do not know how to properly respond by perhaps consoling and displaying affection.

c. Motor skills are underdeveloped

They also have difficulty with motor skills. In a place that requires you to move fast such as in a basketball game, they may not fully understand how to catch a ball. Another example is when a certain situation requires you to run fast, the affected person may just walk slowly. When they walk, the arms may not swing. They may also cry or laugh inappropriately. Another characteristic they may have is an obsessive interest. There is a tendency for people with Asperger's to have a deep interest in a specific task like collecting or calculating.

d. Narrow or specific set of interests

Another instance is when they are having a conversation with a group of people. They want the topic to be focused on them because they just want to talk about their own interests and likes. Their speech is very fluent just like any other professional. They have a more refined manner to them. These people with Asperger's Syndrome tend to become successful in their chosen field of work since they have these exceptional communication and cognitive skills.

e. Displaying Repetitive Behaviors

Further, the affected people also have their usual routine. They are good at maintaining and doing these things. Repetitive behaviors may also be a characteristic of someone with this disorder. One example is finger twisting. Some may say that these people can adjust to a change in their environment provided that you tell them or teach them in advance. However, if it is a sudden change, it may sometimes cause stress or anxiety. They may also have difficulty accessing their imagination and, as a result, they may have difficulty forming a solution to specific problems.

f. Problems with perception and coordination

Moreover, they may also have difficulty with perception. It is either they have sharp or underdeveloped senses. They have a different reaction when they hear loud sounds, bright lights or unusual smells. They may also experience other related conditions such as being extremely active during childhood years and later as a young adult, they may show anxious or depressed behaviors more often. Obsessive-Compulsive Disorder and Attention Deficit Hyperactivity Disorder may also accompany this condition.

The symptoms may also vary according to age. For adults, they tend to manage the symptoms of this condition. They can learn proper social interaction, although there might be some difficulties. They are mature enough to handle and manage the symptoms of the disorder. In fact, many adults with Asperger's Syndrome get married and have children. This is due to their ability to control themselves and build lasting relationships with other people.

Some traits that are typical with Asperger's Syndrome include keen attention to details and focus on interests, which increase their chances of university and career success. Many people with Asperger's seem to be fascinated with technology, and a common career choice is engineering. But scientific careers are by no means the only areas where people with Asperger's excel. Indeed, many respected historical figures have shown symptoms of Asperger's, including Wolfgang Amadeus Mozart, Albert Einstein, Marie Curie, and Thomas Jefferson.

We must remember that not all people diagnosed with Asperger's Syndrome exhibit all these symptoms. Despite all these difficulties or struggles they are facing, they also have many empowering traits, which include the ability to focus, and can possess strong cognitive and communicative abilities. They may be very good in mathematics, computer, science and music. They have a good memory and logic. People with Asperger's are blessed in their own ways.

Points to Remember:

☐ Symptoms vary across people. Some are able to cope better than others.

☐ Some people with Asperger's Syndrome are gifted with extraordinary cognitive ability, which has largely been misrepresented in the media and films. These people are known as savants.

☐ Some people with Asperger's Syndrome are dedicated to their job and can perform very well at school.

☐ Some people with Asperger's Syndrome have a good memory, logical thinking, and exceptional intelligence.

☐ Some people with Asperger's Syndrome are experts in their chosen topic or course.

☐ A person with Asperger's Syndrome typically has difficulty in social interactions, using their imagination, and developing social relationships.

☐ An individual with Asperger's Syndrome may have difficulty understanding non-verbal language and lack modes of empathy due to a lack of understanding social conventions.

☐ An individual with Asperger's Syndrome often display irrational repetitive behaviors that interfere with daily living.

☐ An individual often must do his or her daily routine perfectly, or it may cause temper tantrums.

☐ An individual with Asperger's Syndrome may excel in mathematics, music and logic.

☐ A person with Asperger's Syndrome may appear anxious and depressed most of the time.

Diagnosis

Asperger's Syndrome is a developmental disorder that still has no specific test to determine if a person has this condition. There are key areas when someone can be assessed for Asperger's Syndrome and these areas focus on facial expressions when talking, language development, social interaction, interest in interacting with other people, motor skills and coordination, as well as attitude and level of intelligence.

If you want a reliable diagnosis of your child's condition, you must consult with an expert in the field. You could either go or ask for the advice of a family doctor who can make a referral, psychiatrist, pediatrician, child psychologist, speech therapist or other health experts. If you are the primary caregiver of someone who is suspected to have Autism, you must be very mindful of your loved one's noteworthy behaviors, emotions and personality. Doing so would allow you to work hand in hand with professionals in helping your loved one resolve the issues of his condition. It is of vital importance that your loved one whom you think possesses an underlying condition be assessed, diagnosed, and treated as soon as possible.

The assessment and diagnosis of any psychological condition usually begins with an initial screening. The screening process requires the full attention of the suspected patient's parent, guardian or relative. The background information, family history, as well as eating and sleeping habits are asked. However, this type of screening method is not enough to accurately determine if a child has Autism or Asperger's syndrome. This is why a detailed diagnosis must be conducted to prevent the overlapping of the symptoms of Asperger's with other similar disorders. An accurate diagnosis is very important because it will guarantee that the treatment and intervention programs are tailored to the patient. To achieve this, experts use certain diagnostic tools such as Childhood Asperger Syndrome Test (CAST), Autistic Diagnostic Interview-Revised (ADI-R), Checklist of Autism in Toddlers (CHAT), among others.

Health experts who have little experience when it comes to dealing with Asperger's usually struggle with identifying the defining characteristics of the disorder. This is why consulting with a team of experts (psychologist, occupational therapist, speech therapist, neurologist, and psychiatrist) is ideal in diagnosing children with Asperger's syndrome.

Tips to achieve an accurate diagnosis:

The parents or primary caregivers must work closely with a health professional in discussing matters that involve the suspected patient. Parents and health experts must have scheduled sessions together with the child in order for them to observe his behavior in response to different situations. The goal is to have a

25

deeper understanding of how the child behaves and acts at home and/or school.

In order to rule out or identify medical conditions that require the intake of medication, the child should also see a developmental pediatrician or a neurologist.

Since a lot of people with Autism have poor communication skills, the child's speech and language abilities should also be evaluated. Doing so would allow the parent or guardian of the child to gain additional and valuable information about the condition.

The procedure of diagnosing Asperger's syndrome usually involves a series of check-ups, tests and a comprehensive investigation of the individual before an accurate verdict is made. When a person undergoes psychological assessment, he or she is tested for his or her overall intellectual functioning. His or her strengths, weaknesses, and learning style are also determined through a series of tests. The target areas to be analyzed and measured include his problem solving, motor, perceptual skills, as well as other executive functions.

You must remember that it is never too late to seek for a formal diagnosis. Increasing your awareness about the condition and verifying if someone you know has Asperger's syndrome will significantly affect that person's life positively. Discovering that a person has Asperger's will give the individual and his loved ones an explanation as to why he or she seems to think, behave and act differently. It would also allow them to maximize their strengths and work around the areas of their lives that need improvement.

CHAPTER 2: THERAPIES

Research has shown that acceptable treatment for children suffering from AS organizes therapies that address main symptoms of disorder, which include poor communication skills and also repetitive routines which are obsessive. Medics say that early intervention bears fruit since there is no defined treatment. Applied behavior analysis or ABA and social skills technique training which is impactful on interpersonal interactions.

Diverse researches and studies on the behavior-based in people suffering from Asperger's shows that when the intervention is done early, risks are reduced and data shows that about five people will have little problems later. These intervention programs will reduce self-injury by the patient, noncompliance, aggression, spontaneous language, stereotypes and the unintended side effects. Despite the quality of program of social skills training and, its impact and effectiveness have not been fully established. Results of a randomized and controlled study on Asperger's syndrome with parents and the children who were victims of this condition showed a great improvement in their children when it was done in institutions. But for parent who had received individual lessons told of less and impactful behavioral change among their AS children. Therefore vocational training plays a major role in training these children etiquette and workplace mannerisms. There are also an organization software and even personal data supporters which improve the life and work in the management of adults and children with AS.

In its simplest definition, Asperger's Syndrome is an all-encompassing developmental and growth disorder which occurs mostly in children. The signs of this disease include repetitive tendencies or behavior and a great and impairment in the social interactions among children. It is also known as Asperger's disorder whose acronym is PDD or pervasive development disorder. Asperger's syndrome is named after an Austrian doctor, Hans Asperger. He was the first to define this disorder in1944 but its complexities came to be discovered much later in life through research, observation and much study who first described the disorder in 1944.

It does not come as singular but PDDs are not one condition but a group of diseases that inhibit development through delays of a child's conditions mainly basic or introductory skills. And like said earlier, the child' socialization ability, the power of imagination and the ability to communicate are hampered. Asperger's syndrome is different from autism but it still has similarities with autism which is part of the PDD group but comes as a very severe type. If one has to compare a child suffering from autism with one suffering from Asperger's syndrome, the one who suffers from Asperger's Syndrome has more mobility and his functions are fairer than the one with autism. Children suffering from Asperger's syndrome will always showcase their normal intelligence and at times a near-conventional language development but the challenge with their communication deteriorates as they continue they get older.

Symptoms of Asperger's Syndrome

The indications of Asperger's Syndrome range from modest to severe and may vary from one child to another. Children who suffer from this condition will experience a great challenge when it comes to socializing and interacting with their friends. At other times they will behave in an unconventional and awkward manner when it comes to social gathering. To make friendship for them is an arduous task. They will also face difficulties in beginning and sustaining a conversation. It is this challenge in their social skills that a lot of care and time have to be spent.

Another characteristic that these children depict is their repetitive behavior or strange behavior. They many times develop movements that are repetitive like the wringing of their fingers or at other times their hands.

These children will also exhibit rituals in their own unusual pre-occupancies. The child may develop a habit of sucking their thumbs and do it with a military precision. Any attempt to stop such behavior is usually met with resistance. They could also be engrossed with putting on the same dress and never want to wear anything else. From the symptoms addressed here, one can see that this condition acts a barrier to a child in enjoying life to the fullest with his peers.

These challenges come in multiples with proper communication not well-tailored to give the child the freedom and liberty to socialize. A child with this condition cannot be able to maintain eye contact when he is having a discussion with another person. The situation does not end there since for they also experience problems in use of gestures and facial expressions. And so it becomes hard for them to discern body language. The cycle of challenges that these children face includes understanding language in its real context and therefore they are not able to actualize use of language. These challenges never end with the above.

Their interest range and diversities are at times diminished though such a child may have an obsession in limited areas like the weather conditions, sports programmes and things like maps. Coordination problems are also a major challenge to children who suffer from Asperger's syndrome. Their movements are disjointed, awkward and at times clumsy. On the side of talents or skills, children suffering from Asperger's syndrome are heavily endowed in specific areas like in mathematics and music.

Chapter 3: Compassionate Understanding of the Asperger Adult

Most adults with Asperger's have lived their whole lives without understanding what is wrong with them. Their families have also suffered and lived in confusion. A correct diagnosis can change everything. This "Ah-ha" phenomenon is often accompanied by relief on the part of family members. But with it comes grief when the realization hits home that there is little likelihood of gross changes in the Asperger adult. For instance, the daughter whose son is diagnosed with Asperger may then realize that her father had the same constellation of symptoms, and the reason for her father's apparent disconnectedness, coldness, and inability to empathize with her suddenly becomes crystal clear.

Take this example of a woman who exhibited all the classic symptoms of Asperger. Previous to her diagnosis, this woman had suffered enormously as her husband and kids. The people around her started referring to her as "The Hologram." The explanation was that "she looks like a normal being; smart with a good job, but there is just nothing there." The people around her were constantly trying to figure out how they can interact with her in a way that does not result in stress.

The term "hologram" was an unwittingly apt description of her. There was no intimacy, no understanding, no empathy, just a pragmatic approach to life that did not take into account the emotions of the people she dealt with. Nor was she able to adapt herself to the changing needs of different individuals or situations. The diagnosis of this woman's grandchild with Asperger led to a realization by her own adult kids as to why their mother was the way she was. It answered a lot of questions, and gave these adult kids some closure regarding the childhood hurts they had experienced due to her inability to relate to them.

Dealing with a person with this condition can be extremely difficult at times, particularly when the person has yet to be diagnosed with the disorder. When diagnosis of the adult Asperger occurs, it is often as a result of a child or grandchild being assessed with the disorder. It then becomes apparent to other family members that the undiagnosed adult they have struggled for so long to understand or relate to also have the disorder.

Problems Dealing with an Asperger Adult

Dealing with an adult who has Asperger Syndrome can be clouded by a significant amount of challenges. Some of these challenges include:

A feeling of trepidation due to the effect of this constant vigilance.

A sense of frustration that you cannot "get through" to this person.

A sense of hopelessness that the person doesn't love you.

Depression related to the knowledge that the individual won't get better.

Difficulties accepting the condition.

Failure to understand why the person cannot relate to you in a "normal" manner.

Feeling overly responsible for the person; feeling a need to constantly explain their inappropriate behaviors and comments to others.

If the adult Asperger is a marriage partner, concerns over whether to stay in the relationship are at times overwhelming.

Lack of emotional support from family and friends who do not understand the condition.

Lack of intimacy in the relationship and a failure to have your own needs met.

Asperger makes for difficulties in understanding the emotions of others, as well as, interpreting subtle communication as transmitted through eye contact, facial expressions, and body language. This often leads to the person with this disorder being labeled as rude, uncaring, cold, and unfeeling. While it is natural for those who interact with Asperger to feel this way, it is unfair to the Asperger adult.

This is because Asperger is a genetic, neurological condition which renders the individual mentally unable to readily understand and interpret the emotional states of others.

Many Asperger's adults can maintain ongoing relationships; however, due to their neurological inability to effectively communicate on an emotional level, there are numerous difficulties. Even dating can prove to be a problem as the subtle "language of love" which operates during the courtship phase is often a mystery to the Asperger's individual. This can apply to even the most academically gifted individual. Recent research on the sexual behaviors of Asperger's suffers indicates that they have similar sex drives as the general population but seldom possess the social skills to deal with the high level of intimacy required of such a relationship.

In fact, research suggests that the divorce rate for couples in which one partner has Asperger's is around 80%.

Chapter 4: It A-S How You See It

A major reason why Aspies are often ostracized is due to the disconnect between how they and people around them see the world from very different points-of-view. This leads to one misunderstanding, one miscommunication after another.

What AS may look like to others?

A person outside of the exclusive world of Aspies may take an over simplistic view of AS as cold eccentricity bordering on bizarre.

For normal people, the actions, intentions, words, and reactions of an Aspie to specific situations and people may be seen as indifference. Oftentimes, the things an Aspie does or says can mean one of two extremes---sheer apathy or, overstepping on other peoples' boundaries.

Typical people cannot relate to the secret world only an Aspie shares with other Aspies. There are specific reactions to stimuli people expect from other people during conversations, social engagements, and specific situations. While other typical people will exhibit these expectations, which often are learned easily and demonstrated naturally, the Aspie will do and say things which other people will judge to be rude. Typical people cannot be blamed to expect conformity to norms.

Little do they know, however, that the results of their negative reactions and judgments can be socially debilitating on the part of an Aspie.

Inside the mind of an Aspie

In order to foster a solid, trusting relationship with a family member who has AS, you need to understand what it is behind those annoying noises he makes while everyone is conversing and laughing on the table; why he may seem unresponsive to you; or, why he is reacting inappropriately.

Before you light up your fuse out of annoyance towards an Aspie, take some time to read and understand below some of the reasons why an Aspie behaves the way he does:

People with AS have an inherent physiological incapacity to process and understand stimulus. This is the reason why they do not act or react according to social norms.

People with autism, AS included, are wired to have either hypersensitive or hyposensitive senses of hearing, sight, taste, smell, touch, balance, and awareness. Either way can make an Aspie very irritable and prone to display signs of AS. Below are specific ways an Aspie's senses are stroked by environmental stimuli:

Hearing: Aspies can hear everything. This makes it hard for them to focus and concentrate on just one sound, that includes your voice when you're talking to one.

Sight: When an Aspie looks at you, he is not focusing on your face, and instead may be zeroing in on a mole at the tip of your nose or the lines inside your retina. This makes it difficult for an Aspie to associate a mobile phone, for example, with the word "mobile phone".

Taste: An Aspie's taste buds may either be poorly or extremely sensitive to all the flavors in food.

Smell: An Aspie's olfactory nerves may be too sensitive or, too weak to smell. What could be a mild odor for you may be extremely overpowering for an Aspie.

Touch: You may have seen a loved one with AS inflict pain on him and does not even seem to notice it. That's because he can't feel the painful sensation. Other Aspies, on the other hand, may not like even a light brush on the elbow because that could be very painful for them.

Sense of balance. Aspies have a poor sense of balance, making it difficult for them to participate in any physical activity.

Body awareness. Typical people will normally get mad when an Aspie gets too close for comfort. Aspies do not mean to put others around them in an awkward situation. It's just that they have limited body and spatial awareness. This also makes it difficult for them to perform activities that require fine motor skills, as simple as cutting paper.

Aspies have a tendency to live in solitude. Many, not out of their own will and want to be alone, however. Most Aspies do not reject social interaction rather; they are confused and unsure of how they can relate to other people around them. Peoples' negative reactions towards their seeming strangeness is what drives them to avoid, even despise, social interactions.

Understand that Aspies are inherently incapable of empathizing and sympathizing with others. They cannot recognize simple facial expressions, more so human emotions and other non-verbal hints.

Aspies have a different, unique way of perceiving people and objects around them. Where you see a cold, yummy sundae, an Aspie sees the cherry on top. He cannot see things the way you do. He has a limited capacity to see the big picture.

Even when it comes to understanding people's emotions, an Aspie needs the situation to be broken down into very short segments that an Aspie can digest

43

piece-by-piece. So, to make an Aspie understand why another family member got angry at some action he did, you need to break down the entire situation, discuss it one-by-one with him, and validate that he understands each of these segments.

What it means to live with an Aspie

To live and love an Aspie means you must become capable of living in the world of typical people while keeping the world of an Aspie in sight. There is no other way but to keep a monitor for each rolling in your dashboard all the time.

Obviously, adjustments have to be made. Families and loved ones have a key role to play in supporting positive, significant improvements in the life of an Aspie. Below are some pointers you may follow to support a loved one who has AS:

Know that treatment does not only involve your loved one who is AS-challenged, but so do every other member of your family, and everybody else who cares about him.

Be observant and take notice of his interests and find ways for him to express these. Recognize his limitations and seek professional help. Keep track of things that make him tick so you can help avoid these to prevent signs of AS from manifesting.

Treat an Aspie as you would treat anybody else his age but, try not to impose any expectations, most especially those that call for conformity, so that you do not frustrate him and yourself. When an Aspie falls short of social norms, do not judge. Initially, it will take much effort but, with regularly reminding yourself, this will become natural and habitual.

Develop a routine and stick with it as much as you can. Changes in routines disrupts an Aspie's expectations and may cause him to become upset. If there are items in your routine that you need to change, give him time to cope with the new arrangements.

Do not get too personal or emotional whenever you do not obtain the attention you seek from an Aspie. Whenever you feel neglected, bored or, uninteresting, remind yourself of the fact that your loved one is inherently wired to overlook your feelings and your needs.

At the onset, it does seem difficult to be the person who gives more in your relationship with an Aspie. Over time, not only will your efforts and sacrifices pay off, it will become natural but, don't expect it to ever become easy. Once you build trust and confidence with an Aspie, he can be very loyal to you and it will encourage him to share with you what he thinks and how he feels.

Chapter 5: Effects of the Syndrome on Social Interaction

We have repeatedly mentioned in the previous chapters the problems, inadequacies and difficulties exhibited by the patients with Asperger Syndrome in reference to their social functions, skills and interactions. It's now time to take a closer look at them.

One thing to always keep in mind is that the social interaction problems pertain to the views of the people around the patients and not to the patients themselves. Just as some people feel quite comfortable being around other people, aspies feel comfortable being left alone and at liberty to carry on with their daily routines and interests without outside interference.

One of the main arguments used by the supporters of the notion that those who exhibit the symptoms of the syndrome and present no danger to themselves or others should be considered as merely "different" and not as patients is that the obsession to force aspies into acquiring these social interaction skills is an invasion of privacy. This policy aims not to benefit the aspies but the rest of the social network.

The latest studies on the subject found that both views are actually incorrect. People with AS **want** to interact socially like anyone else. They **want** to acquire friendships as much as anyone else. So it is wrong to assume that they want to be left alone, but it is also wrong to say that teaching them what they need to know about social interaction is an invasion of privacy.

If someone wants to interact socially and have friends, there are some rules and protocols involved that must be respected. When this someone has no knowledge or perception of these rules and protocols, he or she may feel and act out of context. Thus, they need to be shown these rules and protocols.

The first issue that seriously impacts people with AS, not so much for them as for the people of their immediate environment, is the apparent lack of empathy. People who do not know that this person on the other side of the social circumstance suffers from Asperger's get incensed when it comes to the lack of attention they are receiving. Quite commonly, aspies show almost no signs of empathy either towards or against the speaker's side of the story.

When people talk to someone about their problems, their dreams, and their opinions, they expect a response from those to whom they talk. When they do not receive an appropriate response, they lash out against the person on the other side of the conversation, without considering that they may be facing a person who is suffering from a disorder. As a result of this disorder, the person may have no interest in listening to anyone's problems, dreams or opinions. They also do not know how to respond to what the other person is saying to them.

This dilemma leads to difficulty in acquiring friendships, failure to enjoy shared activities in which others participate, and failure to celebrate achievements of other people. This deficiency brings forth one of the main issues of social interaction, which is the "give-and-take" mechanic, or, more scientifically, the ability to demonstrate emotional reciprocity.

The rest of the characteristics, like impaired nonverbal communication skills, clumsy or non-existent body posture or gesturing, and a lack of facial expression, are all results of these two basic concepts – empathy and emotional reciprocity.

A crucial distinction must be made at this point. **Nonverbal communication is not the same as body language.** Nonverbal communication is a concept that supersedes and encompasses body language. The definition of nonverbal communication is the process of communication that uses wordless signals. This includes kinesics (the body language), paralanguage (vocal expressions and qualities), haptics (touch), proxemics (concepts of space and distance), and aspects of the physical environment and appearance. It also includes chronemics, the concepts behind the use of time within a communication, which is usually overlooked by doctors and researchers alike.

For a trained eye, a lot more can be said through nonverbal communication than with a verbal one. There is an entire science called the study of micro-expressions. The professionals of this discipline study the facial expressions in split second intervals to determine characteristics or emotions that are not present in speech. This science is used extensively in politics to determine if a politician is lying or has something to hide. While not everyone has studied and immersed themselves in the study of micro-expressions, some aspects are instinctively observed, as they warn others about the negative feelings of the person displaying them. It is well-known throughout the world that avoiding eye-contact means a person is telling a lie or has something to hide.

The lack of facial expressions and displays of emotions is not so much a problem of showing emotions as it as a problem of not being able to understand how others feel. It is a natural tendency of the human being to trust feelings more than words. When not perceiving or receiving these expressions of feelings, people are less likely to trust the speaker. Consequently, we tend not to like the person who shows no   feelings.

But these are not the only problems that pertain to impaired social interactions. Another basic impairment is the frequent urge of an aspie to engage in a monologue. In this monologue he or she talks constantly about a certain topic in a long-winded speech. During the process, he or she does not interpret or understand that the listener(s) may wish to end the conversation or change the topic. They also fail to recognize and often misinterpret the reactions and feelings of the listener to said monologue. This has also been incorrectly interpreted as insensitiveness or as a disregard of the other people's feelings.

Since the syndrome falls under the general category of mental disorders, in the beginning there were some hypotheses stating that aspies were prone to violent behavior and criminal acts. All the relevant studies dismissed these hypotheses as the findings showed that they are more often the victims rather than the victimizers. All of the cases which included aspies in violent and criminal activities occurred by perpetrators who were suffering from a co-existing disorder in the psychiatric range, like the schizoaffective one.

Further studies and research on the effects of AS on the social interaction sphere, showed that in many cases, children and adolescents suffering from this syndrome can behave normally and exhibit regular social interactions and functionality in a closed environment with controlled conditions. The same aspies, when they were taken out into the real world, where the circumstances are not controlled and are more fluid, reverted to their original behaviors and difficulties.

When this happened, the subjects' analysis and observations led them to adopt a rigid behavioral guideline and to apply what they had learned in awkward ways. This further augmented the problem as the more failed social encounters they had, the more their behavior became rigid and unchangeable.

A side effect of these social encounters may result in an aspie developing a condition called selective mutism. This happens when, within a social environment, they do not talk at all to most of the people present but focus and talk excessively and exclusively to people that they think they can trust or that they like.

This makes them vulnerable to manipulation and should such trust be abused, then they stop addressing other people altogether. They will speak only when they are addressed directly and only about topics in which they are interested. It would not be surprising then, if, in a social environment, they withdrew to a location where they thought that no one would notice and occupied themselves with a hobby or an interest.

Because of their idiosyncratic behavior and the failure of other people to understand their situation, aspies may not respond well to notions such as sarcasm, banter or metaphors. Even jokes are sometimes taken seriously and they may feel insulted without understanding the reason behind the insult.

It is unknown at this time why aspies tend to be especially gifted in mathematics and spatial skills. (Some researchers attribute this peculiarity to nature's tendency to achieve "balance" in every situation.) This actually results in more problems, as these children may consider what they are taught in school as ordinary and mundane, while they themselves have progressed far beyond. Inevitably, this results in problems with the teachers and, later on, with figures of authority.

The last issue to consider in reference to the effects of the syndrome on social skills is that concerning marriage and intimate relationships. In these instances, steps must be taken to remedy the situation for the benefit of the aspie. A lack of empathy and emotional reciprocity is, by default, the opposite of the feelings required for such relationships.

How can someone who doesn't even understand what love is, fall in love with someone else? And how can any "someone else" accept the fact that their partner may show no interest, no love, no empathy and no emotions in return?

Such issues are the basis and the focus of the behavioral therapies that are applied to aspies in an attempt to improvement of their social skills. They can live a normal life, but they have to learn how.

Effects of the Syndrome on Behavior and Interests

One of the most important indications that someone is suffering from Asperger Syndrome is their behavior. This is the one symptom that is always present in all cases, and it has to do with the activities and interests which are pursued with abnormal focus and intensity. Aspies devise a daily routine and then stick to it invariably, and they tend to occupy themselves with a specific topic, a specific issue or a specific object.

At this point, it should be stated that aspies can go through their routines and their interests without necessarily understanding why they do it, or even what it is they are doing. They can collect images of stars, for example, without knowing any additional information about the subject. They do it just because they like the pictures. They can even memorize numbers without even the most basic of understanding of mathematics.

This process usually begins around the age of six. In the beginning, they may be involved in a broader spectrum of interests, but as time passes by, and even though these interests may change, the focus becomes narrower and the interests become more unusual. Sometimes this display overwhelms the aspie's family to the point that they become completely immersed.

A problem in this case is that it's normal, to some extent, for a child to become focused on a specific topic from time to time, and this obsession may pass undetected for some time. This is why it is most imperative to pay attention to body language.

The successful diagnosis of AS includes the behavioral and interest patterns as its core part. This part includes the observation of flapping and twisting, other movements of the hands, and complex movements of the entire body. When these movements are repeated in a fashion which seem more prolonged, natural and symmetrical than the simple nervous tic would, it is often an indication of the presence of Asperger's.

To better understand what the observation should be looking for, nervous tics are much faster, involuntary, and without rhythm or symmetry. The movements of the hands and the body of a child suffering from AS are longer, they seem voluntary and ritualistic, and they have rhythm and symmetrical patterns.

Another integral part of the diagnosis of AS is the lack of imagination. A child is normal when he or she plays "as if." Scientifically, this is called imaginative play: a boy pretends that the car he is playing with is the famous Batmobile, or a girl pretends that her doll is a princess.

Children that suffer from the syndrome prefer non fictitious activities and interests, and they have no wish to watch or listen to fairy tales. If a boy plays with a car, that's what he plays with, a car. Not a Batmobile or a Formula 1. If this kind of behavior is noticed, it is a most definite indication of Asperger's.

Stereotypy is defined as a repetitive motion, stance or sound. It can be displayed as simple motions, like body rocking, or through more complex ones, like self-caressing or marching in place. It is considered a standard issue in people suffering from intellectual disabilities such as Asperger's.

Stereotyped behavior does not necessarily mean that the child suffers from Asperger's. It is a clear indication only. It must be verified by the appropriate doctors, as it has been linked with other medical conditions like tardive dyskinesia, stereotypic movement disorder and some types of schizophrenia.

Stereotypy is also associated with frontotemporal lobar degeneration, which is pathological and not psychological or mental and which occurs in people suffering from frontotemporal dementia. An appropriate examination should uncover an atrophy in the frontal and temporal lobes of the brain while the parietal and occipital ones are left intact. Asperger's is suspected when these issues are **not** shown in the tests.

In all four types of autism, stereotypy is called stimming, as it is hypothesized that it is performed as a self-stimulus of the senses, rather than as a method of expression or counterbalance, as it is in other conditions. This is another one of the reasons that the diagnosis must be correct.

If an aspie is given medication that is recommended for schizophrenics, for example, then his or her behavior will get worse. He or she will also have to undergo a different set of cognitive therapies which will actually do very little to improve the condition.

At this time, we need to address another side of stereotypy. The term also means assigning traits to a class of people and assuming that these traits are always there. Let's discuss what the typical stereotypes about people with Asperger Syndrome are.

They are supposedly unable to do things that require social interaction.

They dislike eye contact.

They dislike using the telephone and prefer indirect or person-to-person means of communication.

They get disoriented and have trouble hearing in social situations where there is a lot of people and noise.

They are easily depressed.

Small talk and intimate banter is out of their league.

They assume that all comments or remarks must be responded to.

Most of the time, they do not care what other people think.

Most of the time, they cannot read the body language of other people.

They may feel rejected and regard themselves as failures if a project or an idea they consider as important receives a mixed or lukewarm response.

Their method of interaction makes others angry.

Facing a frustrating situation, they often respond angrily.

In conversation, they are sometimes tactless or divergent and their language is inappropriate.

When they talk about a topic, they talk forever without pause.

If they are asked a question that is difficult to answer, they remain silent.

This is how the rest of the world has **stereotyped** people with AS. Half of the above are myths, some more are greatly exaggerated and only a few are actually true, falling within the symptoms that have already been described.

This is a clear and indisputable indication that while the general population may have knowledge of the term "Asperger Syndrome," they have insufficient knowledge of the symptoms and how people with AS actually behave. This means that there has to be a campaign of information and education on the subject.

Another aspect of the stereotyping of the aspies as a category of people, is that all the above are **negative**. If the general population wants to attribute stereotyped traits to aspies, why not attribute the following:

Their auditory perception may make them the best sound engineers and quite eligible to work in a recording studio.

Their sensitivity to taste and texture may make them exceptional gastronomes and food critics.

Their eye for detail may be quite beneficial to photography, drawing and assisting architects and artists.

They have no sexism or racism issues.

They are very sensitive to disadvantaged people like themselves and could contribute as mediators or arbiters in disputes.

There is extensive documentation of great innovation and invention from people with AS, not only in tangible subjects, but also in ideas and story-telling.

They are relatively incapable of dishonesty, of lying and of many other negative traits of mankind.

Their memory retention may actually be quite exceptional, especially with numbers, historical facts and past situations.

They may have great powers of deduction which make them ideal for crime investigators.

They may have difficulties in acquiring friendships, but they are very loyal friends themselves.

The problem of societal acceptance of the aspies will be further discussed in the following chapters. As a prelude to that discussion, it is worth mentioning that if one was to distance oneself and conduct a study as an outside observer, he would notice that if a balance was used to weigh the positives and the negatives of people with AS, the scale would tilt in favor of the positives.

CHAPTER 6: ASPERGER'S SYNDROME AND SOCIAL INTERACTION

One of the major hurdles in dealing with Asperger's Syndrome is the social difficulties that come along with it. Asperger's Syndrome affects the mind's ability to interpret the world the way everyone else does, especially when it comes to other people. Simple conversations and interactions often become a chore and thus make both the Aspie and the people they are trying to socialize with unwilling to try to overcome the difficulties. Miscommunication and misunderstandings are instead seen as insurmountable gaps in the process.

One of the more obvious social difficulties is the inability to interpret social cues. The human conversation has evolved over the millennia to include hundreds of unspoken, non-verbal contributions that are universally understood, except by people with Asperger's Syndrome.

Our facial expressions are subtle enough that a dog can read our mood and emotional state in seconds, but have no meaning at all to an Aspie. A raised eyebrow, a crooked grin, a sidelong glance, or even something as obvious as a look of shock or horror could be completely ignored or dismissed. Similarly, body language, except in the most extreme displays, will go unnoticed by someone with an autism spectrum disorder. On the other side of the conversation, the lack of those same cues could be disconcerting and strange to a regular person. There will be a lack of eye contact, seemingly inappropriate body movements, and sometimes inappropriate smiling or frowning. They will stand either too close or too far away while they talk. They will not understand politeness, and will often enter a conversation without introduction or invitation.

Another distinct pattern is a lack of empathy for those an Aspie is socializing with. They will not understand the need or use of an apology, nor will they recognize when their audience is uninterested or bored and trying to find a way out.

There are a few simple ways to help social interactions go more smoothly.

1. Always be direct - say what you mean, mean what you say.

2. Do not count on subtlety in any form. Spoken hidden meanings may be lost, and body language will not register.

3. Be understanding. As hard as it is to interact with them, understand that they're having a hard time interacting with you.

With just these few things in mind, it can make any conversation with a sufferer of Asperger's Syndrome go much better, and hopefully bridge some of those seemingly insurmountable gaps.

ASPERGERS, COMMUNICATION, AND SOCIALIZATION

As Asperger's syndrome has increasingly been diagnosed, more treatments have as a result been developed. Categorized as a form of autism, many with Asperger's syndrome find that it is not as disabling as autism. However, kids with Aspergers do need special help in many areas, so it's good to be aware of some of the treatments that are available. Listed here are some of the better treatments for Aspergers.

Since children with Aspergers have a lot of trouble communicating and socializing, especially with their peers, one important area of treatment is social skills training. Basic interaction skills that come naturally to most children need to be taught to a child with Aspergers. Because of differences in speech patterns, for example, they often need to be taught to speak in a more normal sounding manner. In some cases, they also need to learn to make eye contact and to have what is considered normal body language. These children also have to learn how to understand things like humor, sarcasm, and tone of voice, which they often have trouble with. Treatment for social skills needs to be based on the individual child and their particular problem areas.

Teaching a child with Aspergers these kinds of skills is extremely valuable because it allows them to relate to others better. Nowadays, people often expect there to be a drug to treat every condition, but there is no specific medication for Asperger's syndrome. There are, however, medications that can be used to treat the symptoms of this condition. Children with Aspergers often also suffer from conditions like bipolar disorder and depression. In some cases, medication can help to keep these symptoms under control. People with Aspergers can have a wide range of symptoms, and any medication has to be tailored to individual cases. So, Aspergers can't be treated with a single drug but there are medications available to help with the various symptoms.

If your child has Aspergers, it is crucial for you to learn all that you can about the sickness. As there are new reports and curing options continuously being brought to light, this is a lifelong development, so it's imperative not to assume that you already are aware of everything you need to be aware of. You also need to remember not to take things personally if your child ends up acting out in a particular manner or doesn't communicate with a traditional technique. These are normal signals of Aspergers and the child isn't misbehaving this way to be troubling. On occasion, parents of a child suffering from Aspergers need counseling and therapy of their own; aside from the treatments their child is receiving, to help them face the more problematical phases of this affliction.

There are a plethora of things you can do to help a child who has Aspergers and the specific strategy you utilize should be based on the child's care needs. In most cases, you can find effective treatments to help with the more difficult symptoms. While your child will always be distinctive, there isn't any rationale that says they can't also lead a joyful and prolific life. The healing methods for Aspergers that we've been investigating can assist you in discovering the greatest choices.

ASPERGER'S SYNDROME AND EDUCATION

Asperger syndrome is a developmental disorder that appears in the first 3 years of life and affects the brain's normal development of social and communication skills. Those with Asperger's syndrome display varying difficulties when interacting with others. Some children and adolescents have no desire to interact, while others simply do not know how.

So what should parents/carers look for when choosing a school for their Asperger's Syndrome child, or consider in their monitoring of the school environment?

Children with Asperger's Syndrome cope best in schools with small class sizes. This option is less a reality these days when Education systems worldwide are struggling to survive with less funding and increased consumer demand. However, there are many other procedures and practices you can monitor to make certain your child with Asperger's Syndrome is being educated in an optimal setting.

What can help your Asperger's child at school - Asperger Syndrome and Education?

1. Before the school year starts, take your child to the school for a trial run.

2. Just so they can meet their teacher and learn what their day may look like.

3. This is a good time for you to introduce yourself to the teacher and let them know that you are there to help, providing just a basic overview of your child and what works best for them, as far as you know.

4. Recognize that the teacher will have a number of children to deal with and they want to help your child, but they may need to do things differently than you have at home.

5. Let the teacher know that you are willing to support your child with homework assignments or any other projects that may come up.

6. Be an advocate for your child but don't overwhelm the school or make demands on them that make it impossible for them to care for other children as well.

7. If your child is to be mainstreamed, they are likely going to need aid with them throughout most of their mainstreamed classes.

8. This person will be there to help them with difficult work and also monitor your child for overload, allowing them the opportunity to remove your child from the classroom prior to them displaying inappropriate behavior.

9. Inappropriate behavior in the classroom is only going to make them a target for other children and it will serve them well to avoid that possibility.

FIVE THINGS TEACHERS NEED TO KNOW

1. My child needs structure and routine in order to function. Please try to keep his world as predictable as possible.

2. If there will be any sort of change in my child's classroom or routine, please notify me as far in advance as possible so that we can all work together in preparing her for it.

3. My child's difficulty with social cues, nonverbal communication, figurative language, and eye contact are part of his

neurological makeup -- he is not being deliberately rude or disrespectful.

4. My child is an individual, not a diagnosis; please be alert and receptive to the things that make her unique and special.

5. Please keep the lines of communication open between our home and the school. My child needs all the adults in his life working together.

This is just one of the many tricks, tips, and techniques that you can use to help you Asperger's child at school.

ASPERGER'S SYNDROME ON BEHAVIOR AND INTERESTS

Asperger's syndrome behavior is a disorder that affects the children who have some trouble in their development of languages and communication skills. This is called "Autism Spectrum Disorders". Comparing to other syndrome disorders, the Aspergers is difficult with respect to diagnosing process. Only the males will have trouble in having this disorder. Asperger's syndrome behavior is a kind of behavior that has poor intelligence in communication skills and unable to communicate with others easily. This syndrome has miserable social interactions, compulsions, some speech patterns, and other curious mannerisms. The patients with Asperger's syndrome behavior will often be given a facial expression in practice and will have a hard section of reading the body languages of others.

Some other features of this syndrome include motor delays, ineptness, a limited amount of interests and curious preoccupations. The main reason for this syndrome is the trouble of having difficulties to interact with others and try to demonstrate the fellow feelings to others. The Aspergers syndrome behavior is a neurobiological disorder of one, whose causes are not understood completely. There is no any correct treatment for the Aspergers syndrome behavior, but this can be cured by the parents who are educated in giving their children a good training, an educational interpositions, practice in social skills, communication therapy, psycho-medical aid. The children should be treated with the right ailments with some perfect medications.

The person giving the treatment for any particular children will become his case manager during the assumption. The important thing about this syndrome is to provide aid by many people who are well known to them. The correct problem must be identified from the children and it must be cured as early as possible. The syndrome is very difficult for diagnosing.

The children having the syndrome will require early interposition and moreover, they must be treated with good care by making them involved in educational and social training. The particular stress is placed on social development including the present and past problems in the interaction of having friendships and communication.

After the treatment, the children with this syndrome may not show any development in their language. They will have good grammatical skills and moreover, they will turn good with advanced vocabulary skills as soon as in their early age. They will easily interact with other people and they very easily get good communication skills to have a friendly conversation with others. Children with Asperger's syndrome behavior will gain more and be cured by doing the above treatments and education. After the treatment the children sign with above average intelligence.

WAYS TO OVERCOME OBSESSIONS AND COMPULSIVE ASPERGER SYNDROME BEHAVIOR

Obsessions and compulsive behavior are typical problems linked with Asperger Syndrome Behavior. This is often a hallmark sign of Asperger's syndrome. These children may become fixated on a narrow subject, such as the weather, compulsive cleanness, sports statistics or other narrow concern.

HOW TO DEAL WITH THIS ASPERGER SYNDROME BEHAVIOR?

Ways to overcome obsessions and compulsive behavior:

1. Communication

For example, Asperger's syndrome can be explicitly taught better ways of communicating with others which will lessen their focus on obsession.

2. Cognitive behavioral therapy

3. Medications

Medications that control obsessive behavior can be tried to see if some of the obsessiveness reduces.

In some cases, it helps to turn your child's obsession with a passion that can be integrated into his or her own extracurricular or school activities. A consuming interest in a given subject can help connect your child to schoolwork or social activities, depending on the obsession and the behavior.

ASPERGER SYNDROME BEHAVIOR - ANGER AND DEPRESSION

Part of the problem stems from a conflict between longings for social contact and an inability to be social in ways that attract friendships and relationships.

HOW TO COPE WITH ANGER AND DEPRESSION?

1. Communication skills and healthy self-esteem. These things can create the ability to develop relationships and friendships, lessening the chances of having issues with anger or depression.

2. Anger can also come when rituals can't get accomplished or when their need for order or symmetry can't be met.

3. Cognitive-behavioral therapy. It focuses on maintaining control in spite of the frustration of not having their needs met.

While it is better to teach communication skills and self-esteem to the younger children, communication skills and friendship skills can be taught to teens or even adults that can eliminate some of the social isolation they feel. This can avert or reverse depression and anger symptoms as well as obsessions and compulsive behavior.

ASPERGER SYNDROME BEHAVIOR

Families must, to some extent, learn to cope with compulsive behaviors on the part of their Aspergers child. It helps to learn as much as you can about the syndrome and its nuances.

Asperger Syndrome Behavior

Learn as much about your child as you can and learn which things trigger compulsive behavior so they can be avoided. Some compulsive behavior is completely benign and is easily tolerated by everyone involved. As parents, you need to decide which kinds of behaviors should be just tolerated and which need intervention.

Do you want to know how to...cope with your child's difficult and aggressive behaviors?

Understand what is really going on inside their child's head,

How to help your child to cope better in the community and at school, and much more about Asperger Syndrome Behavior

ASPERGER'S SYNDROME ON SPEECH AND LANGUAGE

The goal of speech therapy is to improve all aspects of communication. This includes: comprehension, expression, sound production, and social use of language

1. Speech therapy may include sign language and the use of picture symbols

2. At its best, a specific speech therapy program is tailored to the specific weaknesses of the individual child

3. Unfortunately, it can be difficult to create a child-specific, evolving, long-term speech therapy plan (1, 3).

The National Research Council describes four aspects of beneficial speech therapy-

1. Speech therapy should begin early in a child's life and be frequent.

2. Therapy should be rooted in practical experience in a child's life.

3. Therapy should encourage spontaneous communication.

4. Any communication skills learned during speech therapy should be generalizable to multiple situations.

Thus, any speech therapy program should include practice in many different places with many different people. In order for speech therapy to be most successful, caregivers should practice speech exercises during normal daily routines in the home, school, and community. Speech therapists can give specific examples of how best to incorporate speech therapy throughout a child's day.

What's it like?

Speech therapy sessions will vary greatly depending upon the child. If the child is younger than three years old, then the speech therapist will most likely come into the home for a one-hour session. If the child is older than three, then therapy session will occur at school or in the therapist's office. If the child is school age, expect that speech therapy will include one-on-one time with the child, classroom-based activities, and consultations between the speech therapist and teachers and parents.

The sessions should be designed to engage the child in communication. The therapist will engage the child through games and toys chosen specifically for the child.

Several different speech therapy techniques and approaches can be used in a single session or throughout many sessions.

What is the theory behind it?

Children with AS not only have trouble communicating socially but often also have problems behaving. These behavioral problems are believed to be at least partially caused by the frustration associated with the inability to communicate. Speech therapy is intended to not only improve social communication skills but also teach the ability to use those communication skills as an alternative to unacceptable behavior.

Does it work?

Many scientific studies demonstrate that speech therapy is able to improve the communication skills of children with autism

1. The most successful approaches to speech therapy include: early identification, family involvement, and individualized treatment

2. There are many different approaches to speech therapy and most of them are effective. The table below lists some of the different approaches. In most cases, a speech therapist will use a combination of approaches in a program.

Asperger's Syndrome and Communication Skills

Asperger's syndrome is a form of autism that is characterized by at least average intelligence or above (IQ=90-110+). People with Asperger's are able to speak, able to express themselves clearly in proper sentences but at the same time have trouble communicating. How can this be possible? This brief article is an introduction to the communication difficulties that accompany Asperger's syndrome.

Pragmatic Language

Pragmatic language is a form of language that helps us interact with people around us. It is not how we pronounce or articulate words and not related to stammering or stuttering. Pragmatic language is the ability to follow a conversation, understand humor and take part in the ebb and flow of chatting and talking with friends, colleagues, and acquaintances. The following things are important attributes of pragmatic language:

Attending to the setting, event, and context that shape/direct social language

Tailoring messages to different audiences

Understanding differences in tone of voice, style of language or formality of language

Noticing the mood, point of view or "feel" of the audience

Respecting turn-taking skill in conversation

Introducing topics in a manner that is polite, respectful and not abrupt

Being able to shift smoothly from one topic to another

Keeping the context of a conversation logical, appropriate, concise and relevant

Attending to and contributing relevant information on a conversation theme

Correcting misunderstanding, asking for clarification when needed

Explaining, informing, describing or stating an opinion

Expressing feelings and emotions, sensations, perceptions

Ability to tell jokes and understand jokes

Ability to use idioms and understand idioms

Ability to understand sarcasm

Ability to use language to persuade

Ability to monitor facial expressions, body language, and gestures

Ability to understand the symbolic or abstract message in proverbs or metaphors

People with Asperger's have difficulty in some or all of these skills and as a result, are often at odds with people around them. When you don't understand if someone is making a joke you may take it personally and feel offended or want to lash out at them in return. If you don't understand sarcasm you will miss a lot of information about the social world around you. If you can't wait your turn in a conversation you will be perceived as a bore or monopolies of conversation.

If you don't understand facial expressions you miss a lot of emotional information being conveyed by the speaker. If you don't understand body language you may use the wrong gestures in social exchange or misinterpret gestures causing you to move away, or move to close or touch when touch is not wanted.

These are just some of the communication deficits of people with Asperger's syndrome. These deficits are real but subtle and it is important for the people who know and work with someone who has Asperger's to realize that they will have difficulty in social conversation and appear odd or unusual at times in the way they use language.

People need to realize that anyone with Asperger's syndrome will have pragmatic language deficits to one degree or another. There are programs that assist people with Asperger's to develop better pragmatic language skills and in return for better relationships with others. There are also tests that can be administered by psychologists and speech and language therapists that assess and pinpoint strengths in pragmatic language. It is important to get help when needed and not let people with Asperger's struggle through life with social language difficulties.

Conclusion

We have tried to give as comprehensive of a presentation of Asperger Syndrome as possible. This is a condition where neither the causes have been uncovered, nor has a definite cure has been devised by science and research. This is a disorder in which patients may be withdrawn, aggressive, impulsive, with restrictive and repetitive behavior patterns, linguistic and comprehension inadequacies and cognitive dysfunctions.

But it's also a condition that could lead to great things; one that can even help patients display significant skills and acquire potential for great accomplishments in life, perhaps even winning a Nobel Prize. This is a condition that counts many notable authors, esteemed mathematicians and distinguished theoretical physicists in its ranks.

Should we call Asperger's a disorder? Or should we comply with the wishes of the people that exhibit its symptoms and call them different? Should we put them under the same classification as homosexuals, as they ask? Or should we consider them as people that need assistance and healing, as their parents think when they are children and they are diagnosed with the syndrome? Throughout the book we respected the term they chose for themselves, aspies, and we have used it in our presentation. We have also mentioned the legal implications that exist should they be considered merely "different," as well as Simon Baron-Cohen's opinion that there are two very compelling reasons that their categorization as patients should remain.

For those who put the right of self-disposition above all else, they should be considered as different. For those who oppose the existence of an "ideal" human standard (probably because of the influence of what happened the last time someone considered certain anthropological characteristics as superior and others as inferior), like an "ideal" configuration of the brain, they should also be considered different.

Self-disposition requires a level of self-awareness and the ability to defend oneself, to be able to distinguish what is right and what is wrong. In a great number of the people that display AS, the case is that they either have no self-awareness at all, or very little of it, and they cannot defend themselves, making them good prospects for victimization, manipulation and bullying. As for the distinction between right and wrong, they have their own criteria, which may vary greatly from what the rest of the world and society in general consider as such.

So it's actually a question of practicality. If they can take care of themselves and present no danger to themselves and to others as the law requires, then their wishes should be respected and they should be reclassified from "patients" to "different." But if none of the above is true or valid, they should be considered as patients in need of medical assistance and supervision.

Neither traditional nor alternative medicine deals with the core problem. If they did, there would be no debate. All that the existing therapies do is address and reduce the symptoms and their common bases: the human brain and its complex functions, neuron connections and input translation centers.

Perhaps the Chinese view of the body and mind as a single undivided entity is a better consideration. Or it could be possible that the way Ayurveda is treating the syndrome is based on a better foundation than Western medicine. Or, the case could be that parts of the truth exist in each different view and by putting these parts together, the different views and philosophies may provide an answer.

In the end, it all comes down to simplicity. **Whatever works is good enough!** It does not matter where it comes from. If the condition is rectified and the aspie can take care of his or her own needs after being subjected to a certain set of treatments, this philosophy is good enough for this specific individual. Another set of therapies may work for another aspie. It will also be good enough for him or her as well.

The final piece of advice that we can offer our readers is that no matter what the choice of treatment might be, it will need three elements for it to work:

1) PATIENCE
2) PERSISTENCE
3) TIME

When there is self-awareness and knowledge of the ailment which troubles the individual, the most imperative aspect of any therapy is that **the patient cannot go through it without BELIEVING that it will be effective**. Going through any therapy under the notion that nothing works and that everything is in vain follows logically that everything will not work and that the therapy will not be effective. However, it's not because it's a bad or an incorrect therapy. It will be so because the patient themselves want it to be so.

In the case of Asperger's (and all forms of autism for that matter), the same holds true for those who are supposed to offer support and assistance, like parents, siblings and teachers. Because aspies may not be self-aware, or have an informed knowledge about their condition, it is their families and friends who must learn to be patient and persistent. It is their loved ones who must communicate the message to the individual with AS. If they are impatient and give up too easily, so will the aspie. That negates the point of the exercise.

Thank you again for reading this book!

CPSIA information can be obtained
at www.ICGtesting.com
Printed in the USA
BVHW040039050621
608823BV00013B/3850